CPR
AED and First Aid

Provider Handbook

By Dr. Karl Disque

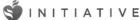

Save a Life

INITIATIVE

Empowered by the Disque Foundation

Satori Continuum Publishing
1810 E Sahara Ave. Suite 1507
Las Vegas, NV 89104

Printed in the United States of America

Educational Service Disclaimer

This Provider Handbook is an educational service provided by Satori Continuum Publishing. Use of this service is governed by the terms and conditions provided below. Please read the statements below carefully before accessing or using the service. By accessing or using this service, you agree to be bound by all of the terms and conditions herein.

The material contained in this Provider Handbook does not contain standards that are intended to be applied rigidly and explicitly followed in all cases. A health care professional's judgment must remain central to the selection of diagnostic tests and therapy options of a specific patient's medical condition. Ultimately, all liability associated with the utilization of any of the information presented here rests solely and completely with the health care provider utilizing the service.

Version 2018.06

TABLE *of* CONTENTS

TABLE *of* CONTENTS

1 FIRST AID

First aid refers to the emergency or immediate care you should provide when a person is injured or ill until full medical treatment is available. For minor conditions, first aid care may be enough. For serious problems, first aid care should be continued until more advanced care becomes available.

The decision to act appropriately with first aid can mean the difference between life and death. Begin by introducing yourself to the injured or ill person. Explain that you are a first aid provider and are willing to help. The person must give you permission to help them; do not touch them until they agree to be helped. If you encounter a confused person or someone who is critically injured or ill, you can assume that they would want you to help them. This is known as "implied consent."

FIRST AID BASICS

The first step in any emergency is the recognition of the problem and providing help. When in doubt or when someone is seriously injured or ill, you should always activate the emergency response system by calling 911. If you're not sure how serious the situation is, the 911 operator will ask you a series of questions to determine the seriousness of it.

Remain on the line until additional help arrives, or until the 911 operator tells you to hang up. Emergency system dispatchers can guide you through the steps of performing cardiopulmonary resuscitation (CPR), using an automatic external defibrillator (AED), or delivering basic care until additional help arrives.

Whether you are at home, work, or school, know where the first aid kit and the AED are kept and be familiar with their contents. Know how to activate the emergency response system (by calling 911 if in the United States). Be aware of any policies in the workplace regarding medical emergencies.

After determining the problem, the next step in providing help is to determine the unresponsiveness of the injured or ill person. The best way to determine this is to tap the person and talk loudly to them: "Are you okay?" After determining unresponsiveness, yell for help. Look for any medical identifications, such as a necklace or a bracelet. This may provide a valuable clue to the cause of the situation.

>> Next: Scene Safety

SCENE SAFETY

Assessing the safety of the surroundings is critical when approaching any scene. You do not want to become another person who is injured or ill so look for any potential dangers. Remove the person from any dangers, such as presence of water at the scene. Be especially alert to avoid danger from automobile traffic.

HANDWASHING AND PERSONAL PROTECTIVE GEAR

Handwashing is essential in prevention of disease and illness. Wash your hands after each episode of care and after taking off gloves. Also, be sure to wash the injured/ill person's hands at the first opportunity. When a sink is not available, use hand sanitizers. (Most hand sanitizers are alcohol-based and are substitute for hand washing when needed.)

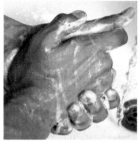

Proper handwashing technique is fairly simple:

- Completely wet your hands and generously apply soap.

- Rub vigorously for at least 20 seconds *(Figure 1)*.

- Rinse your hands with plenty of running water.

- Dry your hands with a towel or air dryer.

Figure 1

Using personal protective gear is an important strategy to minimize the risk of blood and bodily fluid exposure. If the person is bleeding, always wear gloves and protective eyewear when giving first aid care. The universal precaution is to use personal protective equipment whenever there is possible exposure to blood or bodily fluids; it reduces the risk for both the rescuer and the injured/ill person to be exposed to a blood borne disease. Gloves protect your hands from exposure to blood and other bodily fluids while eye protection prevents accidental exposure from splashing fluids.

Consider a pocket mask as part of your personal protective gear as it provides safety during rescue breathing. Be sure to dispose of all equipment that has touched bodily fluids in a biohazard bag when available.

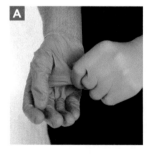 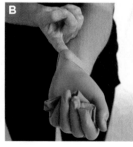 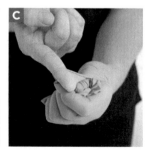

Figure 2

When taking off the gloves, avoid touching the outer contaminated surface. Slowly pull one glove off while turning it inside out *(Figure 2a)*. Place the glove in the palm of the other gloved hand *(Figure 2b)*, and then remove the second glove while turning it inside out *(Figure 2c)*.

>> Next: First Aid Kit

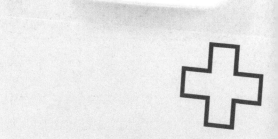

FIRST AID KIT

Consider purchasing a commercially available first aid kit or making your own. Having one available around the house, in your car, and at your place of work is essential.

Common items found in a first aid kit are:

- •Bandages, roller bandages and tape
- • (Sterile) Gauze
- • Antiseptic wipes and swabs
- • Absorbent compresses
- • Antibiotic cream
- • Burn ointment
- • Mask for breathing (rescue breathing/CPR)
- • Chemical cold pack
- • Eye shield and eye wash
- • First aid reference guide that includes local phone numbers

Figure 3

>> *Next: Self-Assessment for First Aid*

1. What is the first question you must ask before you respond to any first aid situation?

    a. Age of the injured or ill person
    b. Safety of the scene
    c. Nature of the injury
    d. Time of the injury

2. Which of the following are considered personal protective equipment?

    a. Gloves
    b. Mask
    c. Eye shield
    d. All of the above

3. What is the recommended amount of time to wash your hands?

    a. 10 seconds
    b. 20 seconds
    c. 1 minute
    d. 4 minutes

ANSWERS

1. B

Ensuring the safety of the scene is critical. Avoid making yourself another injured/ill person.

2. D

Personal protective equipment is essential when responding to any first aid or emergency situation. It is difficult to predict if the person will vomit, is bleeding, or is seriously injured.

3. B

Vigorously rub your hands together using soap and water for at least 20 seconds and rinse thoroughly before and after every episode of care.

>> Next: Medical Problems

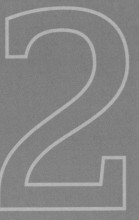

MEDICAL PROBLEMS

Medical problems can range from very minor to life-threatening emergencies. Rescuers trained in first aid must be prepared to respond appropriately.

BREATHING PROBLEMS

Breathing problems can arise from underlying lung diseases such as asthma or emphysema, as well as from illnesses such as pneumonia. Be aware that the other body system problems such as heart attack, stroke, seizure, or anxiety can all result in breathing issues as well.

Signs of a breathing problem include fast or shallow breathing, noisy breathing, producing unusual sounds, or the inability to talk due to breathlessness. Persons with asthma often make a musical sound when breathing, which can be heard as wheezing. Severe allergic reactions can also cause wheezing. High-pitched sounds during inhalation may suggest a partial blockage of the upper airway.

Persons who have asthma or chronic lung disease are generally familiar on how to use their breathing medications. Common medications include albuterol and atrovent inhalers. The use of a spacer (a tube attached to the inhaler that holds the medication until the person breathes it in) can improve the effect of these medications. A person in severe distress may be unable to properly use their inhaler. Call 911 if the person appears in significant distress.

Technique for using an inhaler:

1. Shake the inhaler canister.
2. Place the opening of the inhaler into the spacer if available.
3. Instruct the person to fully exhale.
4. Place the spacer or inhaler into their mouth.
5. Simultaneously have the person inhale slowly and deeply while pressing down on the top of the inhaler canister.
6. Instruct the person to hold their breath for up to 10 seconds if possible.
7. Be prepared to repeat if respiratory problems persist.
8. Stay with the person until the symptoms improve or until emergency response arrives.

>> Next: Allergic Reactions

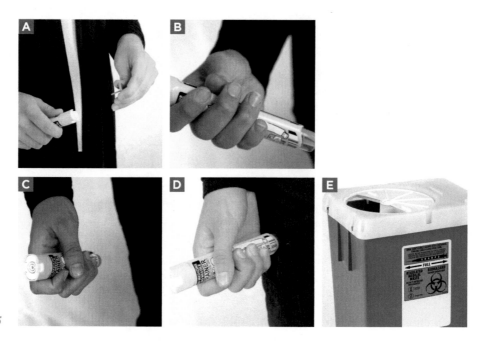

Figure 5

ALLERGIC REACTIONS

Allergic reactions can arise from insect stings, from adverse reaction to foods and medications, or from environmental triggers such as pollens, dust, or chemical fumes. Bee, wasp, or hornet stings can produce rapid and potentially fatal reactions while common food triggers include nuts, eggs, and fruits. Symptoms may be mild, such as itching and hives, or severe causing life-threatening swelling of the airway, lips, and tongue.

Epinephrine can be a life-saving medication and should be given at the first sign of a severe allergic reaction. Commercially available epinephrine pens, such as EpiPen®, are simple to use.

The basic instructions for using epinephrine pens are as follows:

1. Form a fist around the pen and remove the safety release cap *(Figure 5a & 5b)*.
2. Place the orange end of the pen against the outer mid-thigh (with or without clothing) *(Figure 5c)*.
3. Push down hard until a click is heard or felt, and hold the pen in place for 10 seconds *(Figure 5d)*.
4. Remove the pen and massage the injection site for 10 seconds.
5. Properly dispose of the used device in a sharps container *(Figure 5e)*.
6. Note the time of the injection.
7. Seek medical care.

Antihistamines, such as diphenhydramine (Benadryl®), are also important in the treatment of severe allergic reactions. Be aware that epinephrine will wear off, and the persons receiving an injection should be evaluated at an appropriate medical facility.

>> *Next: Heart Diseases*

HEART DISEASES

Heart disease remains the leading cause of death in the United States. Your prompt actions can mean the difference between life and death during a heart attack. If the person is experiencing a heart attack, blocked blood flow to the heart tissue results in muscle death. (Keep in mind the mantra: Time Is Muscle.) Prompt response and medical attention is critical in limiting damage to the heart muscle.

Chest discomfort can be described as ache, pressure, squeezing, or crushing. Certain persons such as women and diabetics are less likely to have classic signs of a heart attack. These individuals may simply experience nausea or unexplained fatigue. Shortness of breath could be the only sign of an impending heart attack for some individuals.

Denial often adds a significant delay in seeking care. Many persons argue that they are too young or too healthy to have a heart attack. Even those with minimal risk factors can suffer a heart attack.

Aspirin keeps blood clots from growing larger and may reduce the severity of a heart attack. If there is no true allergy to aspirin, no serious bleeding, and no signs that suggest a stroke, give aspirin to the person.

When caring for a person who may be having a heart attack, do the following:

1. Keep the person and yourself calm.
2. Have the person sit or lie down.
3. Activate the emergency medical system by calling 911.
4. Give 2 to 4 baby aspirins or half to a full adult aspirin tablet. Make sure the aspirin is not enteric coated.
5. Be prepared to administer CPR. Heart attacks can become fatal quickly.

A heart attack is a life-threatening medical emergency. Persons with symptoms of a heart attack should be transported to the hospital via emergency medical services (EMS). Do not allow a person suspected of having a heart attack to drive themselves to the hospital. Encourage the person to wait until EMS arrives. If they refuse, find someone to go with them.

FAINTING

Fainting is a common reaction to a variety of conditions. Individuals may faint at the sight of blood or during periods of intense emotional stress. More serious conditions, such as an abnormal or erratic heart rhythm, can also cause fainting. Also, severely dehydrated persons may faint when standing up suddenly. The body's reaction to the decreased blood flow to the brain causes the person to pass out. By lying down, blood flow to the brain is improved.

When caring for a fainting person, do the following:

1. Ensure safety of the scene.
2. Help the person lie down.
3. Elevate their legs if possible.
4. If there is no rapid improvement or the person becomes unresponsive, call 911.

A person can also faint while seated in a chair. In this case, help them to the floor. Be aware of the potential for injury if the person has fallen. If the person does not quickly regain consciousness, immediately call 911. Keep in mind that fainting can be caused from a wide range of problems, some of which can be life-threatening. If you are unsure of the cause of fainting, call 911.

>> *Next: Low Blood Sugar in Persons with Diabetes*

LOW BLOOD SUGAR IN PERSONS WITH DIABETES

Diabetes affects a person's ability to regulate blood sugar. Fluctuations in blood sugar in either direction can produce symptoms. Persons with diabetes can experience low blood sugar due to illness, stress, skipping meals, or taking too much insulin.

Low blood sugar can cause altered states of consciousness such as agitation, confusion, and loss of consciousness. Very low blood sugar can result in excessive tiredness, weakness, and even seizure-like activity.

When dealing with a person suspected of having low blood sugar, do the following:

1. Give them a sugar-containing beverage, such as fruit juice, milk, or a soft drink.
2. Encourage them to sit or lie down.
3. Call 911.
4. If their symptoms improve, encourage them to eat.

Glucose gel and tablets are available and are a good way to quickly increase blood sugar. Alternatives to gels and tablets include packets of sugar, honey, or jelly from restaurants which may be readily available. Consider keeping any of these in the first aid kit.

If a person with diabetes is unable to sit up or swallow safely, do not give them anything to eat or drink. This could result in choking or aspiration.

STROKE

A stroke, sometimes called a brain attack, is a medical emergency caused by a blocked blood vessel or bleeding in the brain.

Persons experiencing a stroke will have symptoms that can include the following:

- Slurred or unintelligible speech
- Facial droop
- Numbness
- Weakness on one side of the body
- Difficulty walking or maintaining balance
- Loss of vision
- Severe headache
- Loss of consciousness

Stroke is a neurological emergency, so time is critical.

If you suspect a person is having a stroke, do the following:

1. Immediately call 911.
2. Help the person sit or lie down.
3. Retrieve an AED and first aid kit.
4. Record the time that neurologic symptoms were noted and the last time the person was free of symptoms.
5. Be prepared to perform CPR if needed.

>> Next: Seizures

SEIZURES

Seizures result in abnormal body motion due to an irregular electrical discharge in the brain. Seizures can involve one or both sides of the body. Many seizures result in rhythmic jerking motions, but some seizures may result in a blank stare type of behavior. A person having a seizure may fall to the ground, bite their tongue, and lose control of bowel and bladder. Seizures are often accompanied by a brief period of unresponsiveness.

Causes of seizures or seizure-like activity include epilepsy, low blood sugar, head injury or trauma, heart disease, ingestion of a toxin, or heat-related illness.

When caring for a person experiencing a seizure, do the following:

1. Help them to the ground if needed.
2. Clear the area around them to prevent injury.
3. Place a small pillow or towel under their head.
4. Call 911.

After the seizure is over, do the following:

1. Feel the person's pulse. (Keep in mind that heart problems can cause seizure-like activity.)
2. Position the person on their side to reduce the chance of choking on vomit. (Persons may throw up after a seizure.)
3. Stay with them until help arrives.

Do not attempt to restrain a person having a seizure. Also, do not try to open their mouth or put anything between their teeth.

A victim experiencing an absence or staring-type seizure will have their eyes open but will not respond to you. These episodes are generally brief and not associated with jerky body motion or loss of consciousness. This type of event should be treated like any other seizure and a medical evaluation is warranted.

>> Next: Shock

SHOCK

Shock can be caused by overwhelming infection, blood loss, severe allergic reaction, severe dehydration, or heart problems. When blood flow is significantly reduced, the body does not receive an adequate supply of oxygen, and shock occurs. Victims experiencing shock may lose consciousness or
fail to respond.

Signs and symptoms of shock include:

- Poor skin color that is pale, gray, or bluish
- Dizziness and lightheadedness
- Nausea or vomiting
- Behavior change such as agitation, confusion, or unresponsiveness
- Clammy skin

When confronted with a person in shock, do the following:

1. Activate the emergency response system by calling 911.
2. Help the person lie down and elevate their legs.
3. Cover the person with blankets to keep warm.
4. Be prepared to perform CPR.
5. Stay with the person until help arrives.

>> *Next: Self-Assessment for Medical Problems*

SELF-ASSESSMENT FOR MEDICAL PROBLEMS

1. Which of the following signs is most consistent with a stroke?
   a. Confusion
   b. Chest pain
   c. Facial droop
   d. Nausea

2. You notice that a person has experienced a significant amount of blood loss, has pale skin color, and is becoming confused. What is most likely the cause?
   a. Seizure
   b. Stroke
   c. Low blood sugar
   d. Shock

3. Which of the following is not appropriate when caring for a person having a seizure?
   a. Clear the area.
   b. Immediately call 911.
   c. Protect the person from injury.
   d. Place an object between teeth to prevent tongue biting.

ANSWERS

1. C
   Facial droop, slurred speech, numbness, and weakness are all focal neurological signs that are consistent with a stroke.

2. D
   This is a classic presentation of shock because of blood loss, and it is a medical emergency. Other causes of shock include infection, severe allergic reactions, severe dehydration, and heart problems.

3. D
   Do not attempt to open the mouth or place anything between the teeth. This may result in injury to the person or the rescuer.

>> Next: Traumatic Injuries

3 TRAUMATIC INJURIES

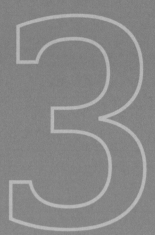

First aid providers are often called to assist with traumatic injuries. Knowing how to respond to a variety of situations is important for first aid providers. First aid responders are valuable in providing initial care and assisting more skilled providers in delivering care to the seriously injured persons.

CONTROLLING BLEEDING

Blood loss often gets the most attention. Many times the amount of bleeding is overestimated and draws attention to wounds when more serious injuries should be dealt with first. Whenever confronted with bleeding, perform a quick overview of the person to make sure something more serious is not being overlooked.

Always use personal protective equipment prior to caring for an injured and bleeding person. The person can be instructed to perform some self-care while you put on your protective gear.

The most effective way to stop bleeding from a wound is to apply direct pressure. Use a dressing and your gloved hand to apply firm and direct pressure to the injured area. Continue to hold the pressure until the bleeding stops. If there are multiple wounds, apply pressure dressings to the worst injuries first, and then to the lesser bleeding injuries. The person may temporarily be able to assist by holding pressure on some areas.

Very small wounds such as scrapes can heal more rapidly by using an antibiotic salve. Ask the person if they have any allergies before applying the antibiotic salve. Thoroughly wash minor scrapes and abrasions with soap and water before bandaging.

Massive bleeding can occur due to extreme injuries such as open fractures or deep lacerations. When direct pressure does not control bleeding, a tourniquet may be required. Tourniquets can consist of a blood pressure cuff, belt, or premade versions. Although commercially prepared tourniquets are more effective than improvised ones, if none is available, one can be made quickly using a piece of cloth and stick-like object. Understand that application of a tourniquet is painful but may be necessary to prevent life-threatening blood loss. Tourniquet use is difficult and can be dangerous if done incorrectly. Direct pressure should be applied first.

>> Next: Controlling Bleeding Continued

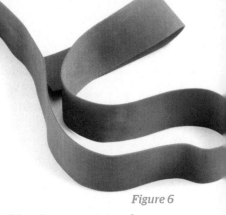

To apply a tourniquet, do the following:

1. Put on personal protective gear.
2. Apply tourniquet approximately two inches above wound.
3. Tighten until the bleeding stops.
4. Record the time the tourniquet was applied.
5. Call 911.
6. Stay with the person and do not release tourniquet until advanced help assumes care.

Figure 6

Certain situations may produce massive internal bleeding that is not visible when examining the person. This may occur from trauma, falls from a height, car accidents, or crush injuries. Penetrating injuries caused by a knife or gunshot may produce devastating internal bleeding with very little external blood loss. Immediately call 911 whenever these injuries are suspected. Help the person lie down and remain still. Check for signs and symptoms of shock. You may need to cover the person to keep them from getting cold. Stay with them until advanced help arrives.

TEETH INJURIES

Teeth may be broken, chipped, or completely knocked out of the mouth. Always use gloves when handling another person's teeth.

Sometimes teeth can be re-implanted and should be transported with the person to the dentist or to the medical facility. Always handle teeth gently and avoid touching the roots. Gently wash the tooth with clean water but never scrub it or its roots. A tooth can be transported in milk, saline solution, or under a cooperative person's tongue. The person must see a dentist or a medical provider immediately.

If a tooth is simply loose, have the person bite down on a piece of gauze and call their dentist. Chipped or cracked teeth can be quite painful. If blood is visible at the crack, prompt dental care is required to prevent loss of the tooth. Injured teeth may later begin to turn color. This suggests an injury to the nerve, and a visit to the dentist is warranted.

NOSEBLEEDS

Nosebleeds can be quite dramatic and are often messy. Be sure to wear personal protective equipment and eye protection when attending to nosebleeds. Persons with nosebleeds often swallow a fair amount of blood, which may result in vomiting. Therefore, you should prepare for the worst.

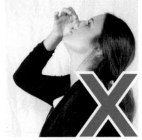

After ensuring that the scene is safe and protective equipment is on, press both sides of the nostrils just below the bony portion of the nose for a minimum of 5 to10 minutes. If bleeding continues, try holding pressure for an additional 10 minutes. If bleeding continues after this, seek further medical care. If the victim has trouble breathing or show signs of severe distress, call 911.

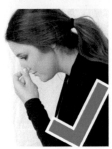

Figure 7

PUNCTURES AND IMPALED OBJECTS

Puncture wounds and impaled objects pose special risk to the injured person. Puncture wounds may penetrate deeper than is apparent and injure sensitive structures such as nerves, muscles, tendons, or blood vessels. Control the bleeding from puncture wounds with direct pressure, and then seek further medical attention. Puncture wounds may carry germs deep within a wound and may result in serious infections. Therefore, any serious puncture wound should be evaluated by a professional as soon as possible.

Impaled objects must be left in place. It is important to understand that the object may pinch off a blood vessel, and removal of the object may result in massive blood loss from an injured blood vessel. Stabilize impaled objects with gauze and dressings and transport the person to the emergency department.

EYE PROBLEMS

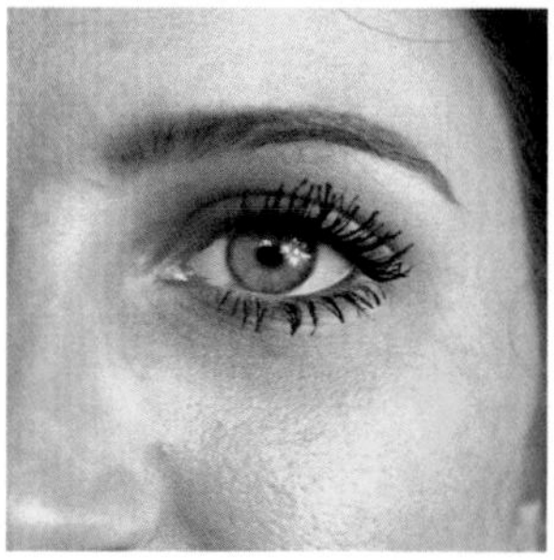

Common eye injuries can result from direct blows, foreign bodies, or inadvertent scratching of the eye. Symptoms include immediate pain, tearing, changing vision, and redness. Bruising and bleeding can also occur. More serious injuries include punctures and lacerations.

Simple irritants such as dust or debris can be flushed using water. Any chemical exposure to the eye should be flushed with copious amounts of water; and you should call 911. Special equipment can be required to adequately irrigate the eye, so you should seek professional care.

Figure 8

If a more serious injury to the eye is suspected, call 911. Protect both eyes with a bandage or eye shield. Because the eyes work in pairs, leaving one eye uncovered causes both eyes to move when the good eye tracks objects. Covering both eyes minimizes the movement of the injured eye. However, doing so leaves the person effectively blind, which can be dangerous and frightening to the person. Never leave a person with both eyes bandaged alone. They will require verbal cues about their environment around them as well as reassurance. A physician skilled in eye care must evaluate these injuries.

>> Next: Head Injuries

HEAD INJURIES

Head injuries can accompany any traumatic event.

Signs and symptoms of a head injury or traumatic brain injury include the following:

- Confusion
- Headache
- Nausea and vomiting
- Memory loss
- Loss of balance and coordination
- Seizure
- Loss of consciousness

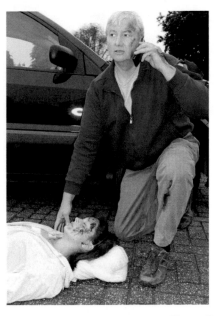

Figure 9

A person demonstrating any of the above should be further evaluated by a physician. Head injuries can be devastating and have lifelong consequences resulting in loss of function and decreased productivity. Permanent disability can occur in more severe cases. Protect the person from further injury by stabilizing the head and neck manually and prepare them for transport to advanced medical care. Observe closely for changes in condition. Be prepared to start CPR if the person becomes unconscious.

SPINE INJURIES

Spine injuries can occur from a fall, diving, car accident, sporting event, or almost any other physical activity. Head injuries may accompany spine injuries. A high index of suspicion must be maintained and efforts must be made to protect against further injury to the spine and the spinal cord.

The following increase the risk of a spine injury:

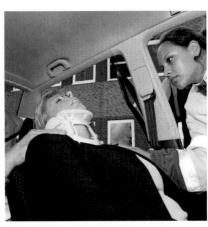

Figure 10

- Age greater than 65 years
- Bicycle or motorcycle crash
- Car accident
- Fall from heights
- Pain in the midline of the neck or back overlying the bony prominences
- Numbness, tingling, or weakness
- Intoxication or substance use
- Other distracting painful injuries

Injuries to the spine can be unstable. Unnecessary movement of the person can result in spinal cord injury and permanent paralysis. When performing first aid on a person with a suspected spine injury, avoid bending, flexing, or twisting the person's head or neck. If they begin to vomit, stabilize their head and neck by placing both hands on the side of the head and neck, and assist them to their side. Maintain stabilization until advanced help arrives. Also, call 911 as soon as possible.

>> Next: Bone and Joint Injuries

BONE AND JOINT INJURIES

Bone and joint injuries are common occurrences in daily life. Physically active people such as those participating in sports are more likely to suffer these types of injuries. The elderly and the infirm are also at high risk for fall related sprains, strains, and breaks. Sprains occur when excessive force or abnormal motion stretches a joint beyond a normal degree. The result of a sprain is pain, swelling, and even bruising. It is impossible to rule out a fracture without an x-ray.

The first aid care for both sprains and broken bones includes the following:

1. Ensure the scene is safe and wear personal protective equipment.
2. Apply gauze to any open wounds.
3. Apply an ice pack to the injured area for up to 20 minutes.
4. Encourage further evaluation by a health care provider and avoid use of the injured part.

Call 911 if any of the following are present:

- Open wound over a joint
- Abnormal position or bent extremity
- Obvious joint dislocation

Consider the following as special circumstances that should be discussed:

An open or compound fracture occurs when the bone breaks through the skin. Do not attempt to push the bone back in and/or straighten the extremity. Bones that are in an abnormal position or bent should be splinted in place. Do not attempt to manipulate or correct an abnormally positioned bone or joint.

A splint can protect an injured extremity. A splint can be made by using magazines, wood, or rolled up towels. Pad the injured extremity, if possible, by using a towel or cloth. Place splint material on either side of the injured extremity and secure in place using tape or gauze. Make sure that the splint is not too tight. The fingertips or toes in a splinted extremity should remain warm and pink. Seek immediate care in a medical facility.

Amputations occur when part of the body is accidentally cut off. Because surgeons may be able to reattach an amputated part, it should always be transported to the hospital with the person.

When dealing with an amputation, do the following:

1. Ensure scene safety, get the first aid kit, and put on personal protective equipment.
2. Activate the emergency response system by calling 911.
3. Apply direct pressure to the bleeding area using gauze.
4. Locate the amputated body part and care for it as instructed below.
5. Stay with the person until more advanced care arrives.

To care for an amputated part, do the following:

1. Wear personal protective equipment.
2. Locate the amputated part.
3. Gently rinse the amputated part with clean water.
4. Wrap the amputated part in gauze and place it in a plastic bag. Seal the plastic bag.
5. Fill up another bag with ice, and place the first bag with the amputated part in the ice bag. Seal the ice bag.
6. Write the person's name on the bag.
7. The amputated part and the person should be transported together to the hospital.

BURNS AND ELECTRICAL INJURIES

Burns can occur from direct contact with any heat source, electricity, or certain chemicals. Burns can vary from minor superficial burns to very deep burns that damage muscles, tendons, nerves, and even bones. High-voltage electrical injuries can produce devastating injuries and can be fatal. Any person sustaining an electrical injury requires an evaluation in the emergency department.

Small burns can be treated with first aid by doing the following:

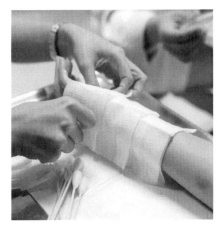

1. Ensure that the source of the burn has been dealt with, and the scene is safe.
2. Wear personal protective equipment, and get the first aid kit.
3. Rinse the burn in cool or cold water.
4. Apply antibiotic or burn cream if no allergies exist.
5. Cover with a clean, dry non-stick dressing.
6. Have the person follow up with a health care provider.

Do not apply ice to a burn. This technique will result in a cold injury on top of a burn and cause further tissue damage.

Figure 11

Call 911 when the following occur:

- A large burn
- Burns on face, hands, or genitals (Burns to skin over joints, such as the backs of the knees, also require special treatment as constant motion will make healing more complicated.)
- Difficulty breathing
- A fire
- Possibility of carbon monoxide exposure

Stop, drop, and roll is the best way to put a fire out from the person. You can also smother the person with a wet blanket to extinguish the flames. Remove the blanket after the fire is out.

When caring for a person with a large burn, do the following:

1. Ensure that the scene is safe.
2. Call 911.
3. Put on personal protective equipment and get the first aid kit.
4. Remove the person's clothing and jewelry if possible.

>> Next: Self-Assessment for Traumatic Injuries

SELF-ASSESSMENT FOR TRAUMATIC INJURIES

1. You are treating a person with a large laceration to the arm. Direct pressure is not controlling the bleeding. What is the next step?

   a. Apply tourniquet.
   b. Go for help.
   c. Start an IV.
   d. Await additional help.

2. A 20-year-old person dove off the end of the dock. Upon reaching the surface of the water, they do not appear to be moving. What is the likely cause?

   a. Heart attack
   b. Low blood sugar
   c. Neck injury
   d. Mammalian diving reflex

3. You respond to an archery range due to an injury. The person has an arrow impaled in their groin. Which of the following is the best option?

   a. Push the arrow through the other side of the leg and remove.
   b. Stabilize the arrow in place.
   c. Remove the arrow and apply direct pressure.
   d. Apply tourniquet, and then remove the arrow.

ANSWERS

1. A

Severe bleeding that is not controlled by direct pressure must be dealt with quickly. A tourniquet is a temporary control measure and could be life-saving.

2. C
Diving into shallow water is a common cause of cervical spine injury and potential paralysis.

3. B
Impaled objects must be left in place. Attempts at removal in the field can lead to uncontrollable hemorrhage and death. Stabilize the object in place. Then transport the person to a hospital for further care.

>> Next: Environmental Injuries and Illnesses

4 ENVIRONMENTAL INJURIES AND ILLNESSES

Our growing quest for outdoor adventures often leads to injury and illness as a result of specific factors related to the environment that frequently require first aid care.

BITES AND STINGS

Insect bites and stings are a common and an annoying occurrence. Most bites are minor but the potential for a serious allergic reaction does exist.

Be alert for any signs or symptoms of a severe allergic reaction, as this must prompt immediate 911 notification.

Bites and stings caused by insects such as spiders, scorpions, and fire ants can cause local reactions, but on occasion more serious systemic reactions can occur *(Figure 12a)*.

Signs and symptoms that suggest a more serious reaction include:

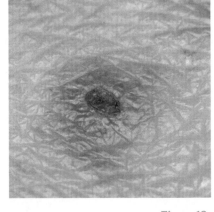

- Nausea or vomiting
- Severe pain at the site
- Abdominal pain
- Difficulty breathing
- Muscle rigidity
- Headache
- Decreased responsiveness

The black widow spider bite is known to cause severe abdominal pain that can mimic appendicitis in children.

Figure 12a

Ticks carry a variety of diseases, and one must be vigilant for signs and symptoms for up to one month after exposure. Signs of a tick-borne disease include fever, headache, joint pain, and skin rash. To remove an attached tick, grasp it by the head with tweezers and pull straight out. Clean the area with soap and water or an alcohol swab. If the tick bite occurred in a geographic area where tick-borne disease occurs, seek medical treatment for possible prophylactic antibiotic therapy.

>> *Next: Bites and Stings Continued*

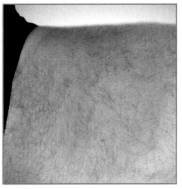

Figure 12b

Lyme disease can produce a distinctive "bull's eye" rash *(Figure 12b)*. Seek medical treatment.

If visible, remove a bee stinger by scraping it away. Wash the area with cold water and apply ice. Stay with the person for at least 30 minutes as some allergic reactions can be delayed in onset.

A bite from an animal such as a raccoon, bat, skunk, fox, or coyote carries the highest risk of rabies. Always make sure the scene is safe when giving first aid to any person with an animal bite. Contact the emergency response system as an animal control officer may be able to capture the animal and determine the risk of rabies. Clean the wound with soap and water and control bleeding by applying direct pressure. Animal bites are prone to infection and can cause further injury due to the puncture nature of the wound. Seek medical care by a qualified health care professional for any bite that breaks the skin, or if there is concern about rabies or other infection.

Snakebites require medical attention. If the pain is getting worse, swelling occurs, bruising develops, or systemic signs (nausea and vomiting) develop, a poisonous snakebite has occurred. Call 911 and do not delay medical attention. Make sure the scene is safe, and the snake is no longer a threat. Keep the person calm and try to avoid moving the extremity that was bitten. Remove any constricting clothing and jewelry from the affected area. Gently wash the affected area with soap and water if available. Additional care is required in a hospital setting. Do not apply a tourniquet.

TEMPERATURE RELATED ILLNESSES

Heat-related illnesses can occur due to extremes of temperature, particularly in the elderly, and during vigorous exercise. Illnesses include heat cramps, heat exhaustion, and heat stroke.

Heat cramps result in painful muscle spasms of the extremities, the back, and the stomach. Sweating and headache may accompany the cramps. Symptoms most often resolve with resting, cooling-off, and drinking water, a sports drink, or a similar electrolyte solution. Light stretching and massage can also be helpful.

Heat exhaustion is more serious. Signs of heat exhaustion include dizziness, vomiting, muscle cramps, fatigue, increased sweating, and lightheadedness.

Immediately move the person to a cooler environment if possible. Have the person lie down and loosen or remove as much clothing as possible. Use cool water to spray them and fan if available. A cool damp cloth can be used as an alternative. Encourage them to drink water or a sports drink. Remain with them until the emergency medical response arrives.

Heat stroke is life-threatening, and immediate action is required. Signs and symptoms of heat stroke include confusion, loss of consciousness, dizziness, muscle cramps, vomiting, and seizures. If you think the person is having a heat stroke, immediately call 911.

When treating a person with heat stroke, immediately do the following:

1. Assess scene safety, wear protective equipment, and obtain first aid kit and AED.
2. Use a spray bottle with cold water and a fan, if available, as rapid cooling is imperative.
3. If the person is able, encourage them to drink water, a sports drinks, or an electrolyte solution.
4. Continue to cool the person until their behavior returns to normal or until advanced help arrives.

>> Next: Sunburn

SUNBURN

Exposure to the UV radiation from sunlight can result in sunburn. Sunburn can be minor or result in blistering and sloughing *(Figure 13)* of skin. Avoidance of additional sun exposure is key. Encourage hydration and drinking of extra fluids. Topical aloe vera can provide symptomatic relief. If not allergic, ibuprofen can also help alleviate some of the discomfort.

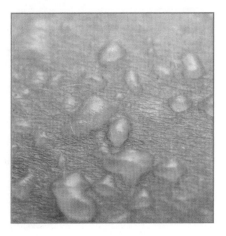

Figure 13

FROSTBITE

Exposure to cold can result in frostbite and is most common in extremities such as ears, nose, fingers and toes. Wind chill increases the risk of frostbite. In severe frostbite cases, ice crystals form in the tissues and destroy cells resulting in permanent damage. The skin will appear waxy and white or yellow-gray. The area will be cold and numb and may feel like a block of wood. The tissue will be firm and will not move or compress easily when squeezed.

To provide first aid for frostbite, do the following:

1. Get the person to a warm place.
2. Call 911.
3. Remove any constricting clothing and all jewelry from the affected body part.
4. Remove all wet clothing.
5. Redress in dry, warm clothing and cover with a heavy blanket.
6. The frostbitten extremity should be quickly rewarmed in hot water (104°F).

Do not rub, squeeze, or slap the affected extremity as this may increase tissue damage. Do not rewarm a frozen extremity if there is a risk of refreezing. Seek further care from a health care professional.

>> Next: Hypothermia

HYPOTHERMIA

Hypothermia is a potentially life-threatening condition when the body temperature falls dangerously low. Hypothermia can even develop in non-freezing temperatures.

Signs and symptoms of hypothermia are:

- Behavior change (confusion or lethargy)
- Paradoxical undressing
- Shivering (but stops as hypothermia worsens)
- Muscle stiffness
- Cold skin
- Decreased respiratory effort
- Progression to unresponsiveness and death

Rapid action is required to care for a hypothermic person.

Call 911 immediately and do the following:

1. Remove the person from the cold and get them to a warm environment.
2. Remove any wet clothing and dry the person.
3. Redress in dry, warm clothing and cover with a blanket.
4. Cover the head as it is a source of significant heat loss.
5. Be prepared to perform CPR. Stay with the person until advanced help arrives.

TOXIN AND POISON EXPOSURE

The list of toxins and potential poison exposures is extensive and beyond the scope of this handbook. Some basic concepts that are universally applicable for first aid providers are included in this handbook.

A material safety data sheet (MSDS) is required to be available where chemicals are in use in businesses and institutions. The data sheets provide information about the composition of various chemicals and are useful when contacting poison control.

To provide first aid in these situations, do the following:

1. Call 911.
2. Ensure the scene is safe and wear personal protective equipment.
3. Get the first aid kit and the AED.
4. Tell the dispatcher the chemicals involved if possible.
5. Remove the person from the toxin or poison and seek a well-ventilated area if possible.
6. Remove saturated clothing if present.
7. Follow any recommendations from the 911 dispatcher or the MSDS sheet.
8. Stay with the person until advanced help arrives.
9. If CPR is required, ensure a mask is used if possible.

When treating any toxin and poison exposures, the eyes should be flushed with copious amounts of water. Acids and alkaline solutions are particularly caustic and can lead to permanent vision impairments or loss.

>> *Next: Self-Assessment for Environmental Injuries and Illnesses*

SELF-ASSESSMENT FOR ENVIRONMENTAL INJURIES AND ILLNESSES

1. A child was bitten by something and now complains of severe abdominal pain. What is most likely the cause?

   a. Black widow spider
   b. Hornet sting
   c. Fire ant
   d. Tick

2. You are treating a person with a frostbite. What is the best way to warm up their feet?

   a. Soak in hot water.
   b. Rub vigorously.
   c. Slap and then massage.
   d. Soak in room temperature water.

3. A factory worker is sprayed in the face by an unknown chemical. Which of the following actions is time critical?

   a. Contacting their personal physician
   b. Having them sit down
   c. Copious irrigation of the eyes
   d. Prophylactic CPR

ANSWERS

1. A

Black widow spider bites can produce systemic signs and symptoms. A rigid abdomen is classic for this type of poisonous bite in children and can even mimic acute appendicitis.

2. A
Soak the affected extremity in hot water of approximately 104 °F. Avoid rubbing, slapping, squeezing, or vigorously massaging as this may cause further tissue damage.

3. C
The eyes should be flushed with copious amounts of water when a chemical exposure occurs. Acids and alkaline solutions are particularly caustic and can lead to permanent vision impairments or loss.

>> Next: Adult CPR, AED and Choking

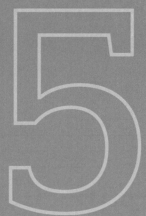

ADULT CPR, AED AND CHOKING

CPR is a vital and an essential skill that can save someone's life. The two key elements of CPR are pressing on the chest, also called compressions, and providing breaths. Any child past puberty is treated with adult CPR. Young children and infants require special considerations for CPR.

ADULT CPR

CPR is comprised of chest compressions, airway management, and rescue breathing. To deliver high-quality CPR, you must begin high-quality chest compressions quickly, as these are considered the most important factor in giving the person a chance to recover. Compressing the chest circulates blood to the brain and the heart. High-quality chest compressions are delivered at a rate between 100 to 120 beats per minute and at a depth between 2 to 2.4 inches (5 to 6 cm).

When the person is unresponsive and is not breathing or only gasping for air, provide CPR. 2017 updates recommend for adults in out-of-hospital cardiac arrest (OHCA), that untrained lay rescuers should provide chest compression only CPR with or without dispatcher assistance. For lay rescuers trained in chest compression only CPR, it is recommended that they provide chest compression only CPR for adults in CPR. For lay rescuers trained in CPR using chest compressions and ventilation, rescue breaths, it is reasonable to provide ventilation, rescue breaths, and chest compressions for the adult in OHCA.

For adult CPR, do the following:

1. Make sure the scene and area around the person is safe.
2. Tap the person and talk loudly: "Are you okay?"
3. Yell for help. Use a cellphone to call 911 and send a bystander to get an AED.
4. Check the person's breathing.
5. If the person is not responding, breathing, or only gasping, start CPR.
6. Give 30 compressions at a rate of 100 to 120 beats per minute and at a depth between 2 to 2.4 inches (5 to 6 cm). Let the chest rise back up before you start your next compression.
7. Open the airway and give two breaths.

Continue giving compressions and breaths until the AED arrives, until advanced help arrives and assumes care, or until the person begins to respond.

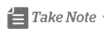 *Take Note*

As a rescuer, if you are untrained in CPR, then give the "hands-only" CPR. The "hands-only" CPR is when you give continuous compressions but no breaths.

>> Next: Compressions

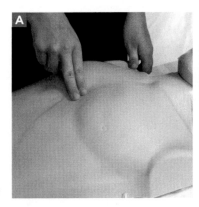
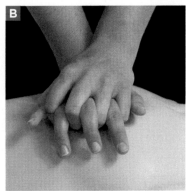
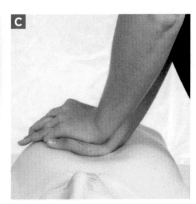

Figure 14

COMPRESSIONS

Chest compressions have the greatest impact for survival. Many rescuers fail to push hard or fast enough. High-quality chest compressions have the greatest chance to save a life.

Chest compressions should always be given at a rate of 100 to 120 beats per minute and at a depth between 2 to 2.4 inches (5 to 6 cm). Compressing the chest slower than 100 beats per minute is less likely to provide enough circulation to the brain, heart, and other vital organs, while compressing faster than 120 beats per minute does not provide enough time for the heart to fill between each compression, which will reduce output as well. Similarly, pressing the chest deeper than 2.4 inches (6 cm) increases the risk of injuring the person, while not pressing deep enough will not squeeze the heart enough to provide adequate blood flow.

CPR always begins with compressions before administering breaths. Rescuers who are uncomfortable performing mouth-to-mouth and do not have a mask may perform hands-only CPR and give compressions at a rate of 100 to 120 beats per minute and at a depth between 2 to 2.4 inches (5 to 6 cm).

For chest compressions, do the following:

1. Position the person on their back on a firm, flat surface.
2. Remove or open up clothing at the neck and chest area.
3. Feel for the end of the breastbone (sternum). *(Figure 14a)*
4. Place the heel of one hand on the lower half of the breastbone. Avoid pressing down on the very end of the breastbone as the bony tip, called the xyphoid process, may break off and slash the liver, resulting in internal bleeding. Put the other hand on top of the first. *(Figure 14b)*
5. Press straight down at a rate of 100 to 120 beats per minute and at a depth between 2 to 2.4 inches (5 to 6 cm). *(Figure 14c)*
6. Let the chest recoil completely between compressions. Your hands should remain in contact with the person, without bouncing or leaning on the person.

Performing proper CPR is often tiring. Ask to switch positions when tired if another rescuer is available to help. Monitor each other's performance, providing encouragement and offering to switch when fatigue sets in.

>> Next: Giving Breaths

GIVING BREATHS

Giving breaths during CPR can help maintain a supply of oxygen in the lungs. Oxygen, in turn, is circulated to the brain and to the vital organs by chest compressions. The preferred method is to use a mask; however, mouth-to-mouth can also be performed. A correctly executed breath will cause the person's chest to rise.

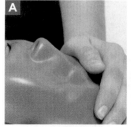
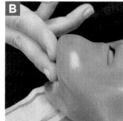
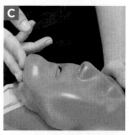
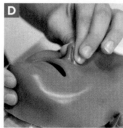
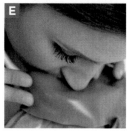

Figure 15

To open the person's airway, do the following:

1. Put one hand on their forehead *(Figure 15a)*.
2. Place your fingers on the bony part of their chin *(Figure 15b)*.
3. Gently tilt the head back while lifting the chin *(Figure 15c)*.

Now you are ready to give breaths. Do the following:

1. Hold the person's airway open as described above and pinch their nose shut *(Figure 15d)*.
2. Take a deep breath and seal your mouth around the person's mouth *(Figure 15e)*.
3. Blow into their mouth for one second and watch their chest rise.
4. Repeat with a second breath.

If the chest does not rise, reposition the airway. Let their head go back to a normal position and repeat the head-tilt/chin-lift maneuver. Then give another breath and look for the chest to rise.

Perform the chest compressions without interruption. It should take no longer than 10 seconds to give two breaths. If the person's chest fails to rise within 10 seconds, begin chest compressions again.

MASK USE

CPR, including giving breaths, is generally safe. If a mask is available, it should be used. The mask fits over the victim's mouth and nose. Most masks have a pointed end, which should go over the bridge of the person's nose.

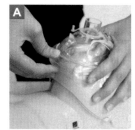
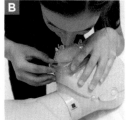

Figure 16

When using a mask to give breaths, do the following:

1. Place the mask over the person's mouth and nose *(Figure 16a)*.
2. Open their airway by performing the head-tilt/ chin-lift maneuver.
3. Ensure a good seal between the mask and the person's face.
4. Give a breath for over one second and watch the chest rise *(Figure 16b)*.
5. Deliver the second breath.

>> Next: AED for Adults

AED FOR ADULTS

When the heart does not work properly, a person may collapse. An AED can deliver a shock to help restart the heart. These portable units have a computer that analyzes the heart rhythm and determines if a shock is needed. Starting CPR immediately and quickly using an AED improves the chances of survival.

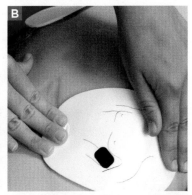
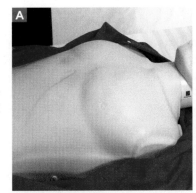

The AED is very simple to use. Follow the diagram or voice instructions given by the AED. Apply the pads properly and let the computer determine if and when a shock is needed. Make sure no one is touching the person if the AED advises you to push the shock button. If an AED is not quickly available, begin CPR and send someone to locate an AED.

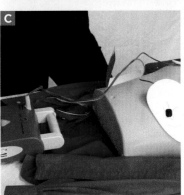
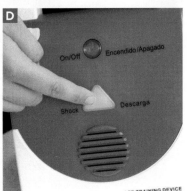

Figure 17

An AED should be used anytime a person collapses, fails to respond and is only gasping, or barely breathing. Turn on the AED and then follow the prompts you see and hear.

TO USE AN AED, DO THE FOLLOWING:

1. Turn the power on.
2. Expose the chest *(Figure 17a)*.
3. Apply pads on the victim *(Figure 17b)*.
4. Connect the pads.
5. Clear the person *(Figure 17c)*.
6. Analyze the rhythm.
7. Follow the prompts *(Figure 17d)*:
   Shock Advised, No Shock Advised, Check Connection, etc.
8. Resume CPR with compressions.

Take Note

If a person has a medication patch on their chest, remove it before applying the AED pads. Also, if there is a bulge under the skin of their chest, a pacemaker may be present. Avoid placing the AED pads over this device and adjust placement accordingly. If the AED malfunctions or does not work, continue performing CPR until additional help arrives.

>> *Next: Activating EMS*

ACTIVATING EMS (CALLING 911)

When encountering a person who is unresponsive, barely breathing, or not breathing quickly, call 911. Immediate activation of EMS by dialing 911 or the appropriate emergency number is the first step in the Chain of Survival. When available, use of a cellular phone may allow activation of EMS without leaving the person. Many cellular phones incorporate a speakerphone function, which allows a lone rescuer to communicate with the 911 operator while delivering care to the person.

In situations where a cell phone is not available, it is preferred to send a second rescuer or a bystander to call 911, so the injured/ill person is not left alone. That second rescuer or bystander may also retrieve an AED and/or a first aid kit.

Always make sure the scene is safe when approaching an injured/ill person. If you become injured or disabled, you will be unable to help the person and will become a second person to be taken care of by rescuers.

Tap the person and talk loudly: "Are you okay?" If they fail to respond or react, they are considered unresponsive. Yell for help and send somebody to call 911 and get an AED if possible.

Stay on the phone until the 911 operator tells you it is okay to hang up. The operator can help you make decisions and will not delay the arrival of additional help.

After determining that the person is unresponsive, check their breathing. If they are barely breathing or only gasping, begin CPR. Gasping may be forceful or weak, but it is generally ineffective. This is an abnormal sign and often occurs in cardiac arrest. In this situation, immediately begin CPR.

If the person is breathing normally but not responding, roll them onto their side. This can help keep their airway open and prevent them from choking on vomit. You need to monitor their breathing and be prepared to start CPR if their condition worsens.

CHOKING IN ADULTS

Choking is a preventable cause of death that occurs when food or another object gets stuck in the throat. The airway gets blocked and immediate action is needed. The person typically only has a few minutes before they pass out. The universal sign of choking is holding the neck with one or both hands.

Choking can be mild or severe. Table 1 will help determine whether it is mild or severe.

DEGREE OF OBSTRUCTION	RESPONSIVENESS	RESCUERS ACTIONS
Mild Obstruction	• *Breathing but may also be wheezing* • *Coughing and making noise*	• *Stay with the person, try to keep them calm* • *Encourage them to cough* • *Call 911 if the person does not clear the obstruction or seems to be getting worse*
Severe Obstruction	• *Clutching the neck (universal sign of choking)* • *Weak or no cough* • *Unable to make noise or talk; may make high-pitched noise* • *Little or no breathing* • *Appears cyanotic (blue around lips and fingertips)*	• *Use abdominal thrusts (Heimlich maneuver) to attempt to remove obstruction* • *Call 911* • *Begin CPR if person becomes unresponsive*

Table 1

>> *Next: Relief of Choking*

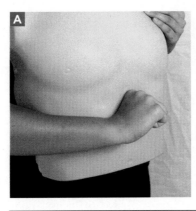
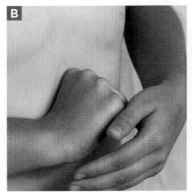
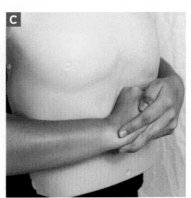

Figure 18:
Heimlich Maneuver

RELIEF OF CHOKING

Abdominal Thrusts (Heimlich Maneuver)

The Heimlich maneuver is used on adolescents and adults.

To perform the Heimlich maneuver, do the following:

1. Stand behind the person and wrap your arms around their waist under the ribcage *(Figure 18a)*.

2. Put your fist above the person's navel in the middle of the belly *(Figure 18b)*.

3. With your other hand, hold the first fist and press forcefully into the abdomen and up toward their chest *(Figure 18c)*.

4. Continue performing thrusts until the obstruction is relieved or until the person becomes unresponsive. If the person becomes unresponsive, begin CPR.

Very large persons or pregnant women can be treated with chest thrusts. In this case, do the following:

Wrap both arms around the person, similar to the Heimlich maneuver. Pull your arms straight back to deliver the chest thrusts. If a person has passed out due to choking, help them to the ground. Use the heel of one hand to perform abdominal thrusts above the navel. Continue this until the food or object comes out or until advanced help arrives.

>> Next: Self-Assessment for Adult CPR, AED & Choking

SELF-ASSESSMENT FOR ADULT CPR, AED AND CHOKING

1. What age is considered an adult for CPR purposes?

    a. Two years
    b. Four years
    c. Six years
    d. Puberty and older

2. You are first on scene and the victim is unresponsive, pulseless and has vomited. You do not feel comfortable performing mouth-to-mouth ventilation. What is the best approach?

    a. Wipe off the face or cover with a shirt
    b. Compression only CPR
    c. Go and get help
    d. Do not initiate resuscitation

3. When are breaths given?

    a. After EMS arrives.
    b. Before compressions
    c. With compressions
    d. After compressions

4. You are performing single person CPR. The AED advises a shock. After the shock is delivered what is the next immediate step?

    a. Call for help
    b. Resume CPR with chest compressions
    c. Check for a pulse
    d. Resume ventilation

5. A college student turns blue and collapses while eating chicken wings at a bar. What is the most likely cause?

    a. Cardiac arrest
    b. Alcohol poisoning
    c. Choking
    d. Drug ingestion

>> Next: Self-Assessment Answers

ANSWERS

1. D

   Any person who is at puberty or older is considered an adult for CPR purposes.

2. B

   Compression only CPR has been shown to be effective. Leaving the victim significantly increases mortality.

3. D

   Chest compressions are always given first. Breaths are performed afterwards. Give two breaths for every 30 chest compressions.

4. B

   Do not stop to check a pulse after a shock is delivered. 911 or EMS should have already been summoned.

5. C

   The color change suggests that they are choking. Patients who are intoxicated are at an increased risk of choking and aspirating food contents.

>> Next: Child CPR, AED and Choking

6 CHILD CPR, AED AND CHOKING

Children have breathing difficulties more often than they have actual heart problems. Therefore, it is important to begin CPR quickly and perform five sets of CPR before going to get additional help. One set of CPR consists of 30 compressions and two breaths.

If someone else is available, send them to call 911 and to find an AED. When they return, have them follow the AED prompts, apply AED pads, and help with CPR.

If the child is unresponsive and not breathing or only gasping for air, provide CPR.

When giving CPR to a child, do the following:

1. Make sure the scene and area around the child is safe.
2. Tap the child and talk loudly: "Are you okay?"
3. Yell for help.
4. Check breathing.
5. If not responding and not breathing or only gasping, then give five sets of 30 compressions and two breaths.
6. Call 911 and get an AED.
7. Resume CPR and give compressions and breaths.

CHILD CPR (1 YEAR TO PUBERTY)

CPR in children is very similar to CPR in adults. The main goals are early administration of CPR, pushing hard and fast on the chest, and giving breaths. Individuals older than one year of age but have not yet reached puberty are considered children. Some children appear adult-size and can be treated as adults for the purposes of CPR.

The term "unresponsive" or "not responding" includes any child who does not move, blink, speak, make a sound, or otherwise react to your efforts to awaken them.

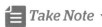 **Take Note**

As a rescuer, if you are untrained in CPR, then give the "hands-only" CPR. The "hands-only" CPR is when you give continuous compressions but no breaths.

>> Next: Compressions

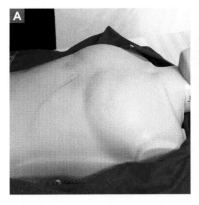
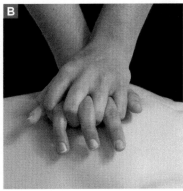
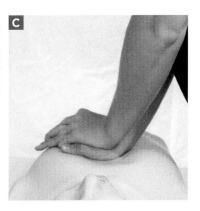

Figure 19

COMPRESSIONS

Rescuers may be afraid to perform chest compressions out of fear of hurting the child. It is important to remember that without CPR, the result will be death.

To do CPR on a child, do the following:

1. Position the child on their back on a firm, hard surface.
2. Move any clothing away from the chest.
3. Place the heel of one hand on the lower half of the breastbone *(Figure 19)*.
4. Push straight down approximately at least one third the depth of the chest. In most children this will be about two inches (5 cm). Compressions should be delivered at a rate of 100 to 120 beats per minute.
5. Let the chest recoil to its normal position after every compression.

Either one-handed or two-handed compressions can be used in child CPR. *(Figures 19a & 19b)* Performing CPR can be tiring. If someone is available to help, change roles every two minutes and work to minimize the pause in between compressions.

>> Next: Giving Breaths

GIVING BREATHS

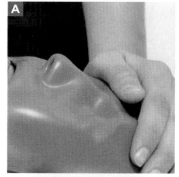
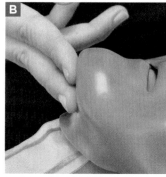
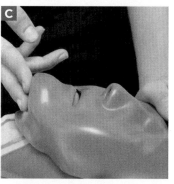
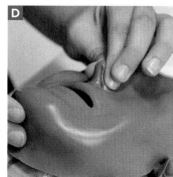
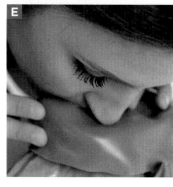

Figure 20

Unresponsiveness in children is often caused by breathing problems, not heart problems. Prevention of choking or severe breathing problems due to untreated illness is the most effective treatment. Giving breaths during CPR can help the child. Severe breathing problems from a respiratory illness can cause cardiac arrest in children. Most children who need CPR have had a breathing problem that caused the heart to beat irregularly or to stop beating altogether.

Signs of ineffective breathing include slow breathing, very shallow or sporadic breathing, and absence of any breaths altogether. Give rescue breaths to children who appear to be struggling to breathe. A good breath will cause the child's chest to rise.

To open the child's airway, do the following:

1. Put one hand on their forehead *(Figure 20a)*.

2. Place your fingers on the bony part of their chin *(Figure 20b)*.

3. Gently tilt the head back while lifting the chin *(Figure 20c)*.

Now you are ready to deliver breaths. Do the following:

1. Hold the child's airway open as described above and pinch the nose shut *(Figure 20d)*.
2. Take a deep breath and seal your mouth around the child's mouth *(Figure 20e)*.
3. Gently exhale into their mouth for one second using enough force to cause the chest to rise.
4. Repeat for a second breath.

>> Next: Mask Use

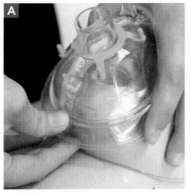
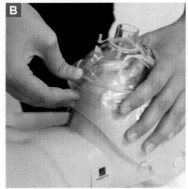
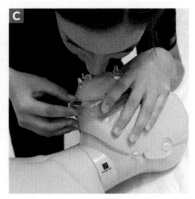

Figure 21

MASK USE

Giving breaths in CPR is generally safe. However, if a mask is available, it should be used. The mask fits over the child's mouth and nose. Many masks have a pointed end, which should go over the bridge of the nose. Make sure the mask fits properly; if it is too large, a proper seal cannot be obtained and efforts to deliver breaths will be ineffective.

When using a mask to give breaths, do the following:

1. Place the mask over the child's mouth and nose *(Figure 21a)*.
2. Open the airway by performing the head-tilt/chin-lift maneuver *(Figure 21b)*.
3. Ensure a good seal between the mask and the face.
4. Give a breath for more than one second and watch the chest rise *(Figure 21c)*.
5. Deliver the second breath.

>> Next: AED for Children

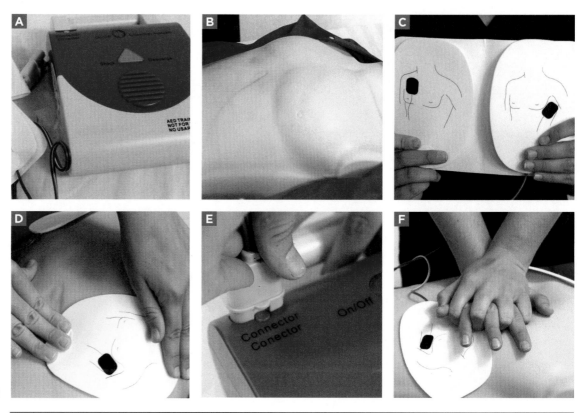

Figure 22

AED FOR CHILDREN

An AED can be used on children and should be used as early as possible but should not interfere with CPR. The steps for using an AED on a child are the same as those in an adult. Check the AED when it arrives on the scene. If the child is younger than eight years, pediatric pads should be used *(Figure 22a)*. Standard (adult) pads may be used if pediatric pads are not available. If using standard pads, do not let the pads overlap each other. You may need to put one of the pads on the child's back if the child is small.

Some AEDs have a switch that can be set to deliver a pediatric shock. If available, turn this switch on when using for children younger than eight years. If the AED cannot deliver a pediatric shock, an adult shock should be given. Be sure to start CPR. If using adult pads on a child, be sure that the pads do not touch.

To use an AED on a child, do the following:

1. Turn the power on.
2. Expose the chest *(Figure 22b)*.
3. Apply pads on the child. Ensure that the pads do not touch *(Figure 22c, Figure 22d)*.
4. Connect the pads *(Figure 22e)*.
5. Clear the child.
6. Analyze the rhythm.
7. Follow the prompts: Shock Advised, No Shock Advised, Check Connection, etc. *(Figure 22e)*.
8. Resume CPR with compressions.

>> Next: Activating EMS

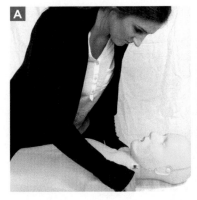
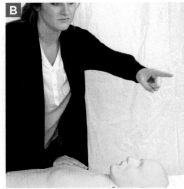
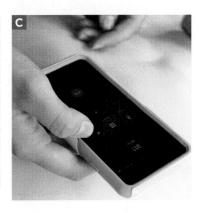

Figure 23

ACTIVATING EMS (CALLING 911)

Always make sure that the scene is safe when approaching a child. If you become injured or disabled, it will only make the situation worse.

Tap the child and talk loudly: "Are you okay?" *(Figure 23a)* If they fail to make any response, they are considered unresponsive. Yell for help and send somebody to call 911 and to get an AED if possible *(Figure 22b)*.

After determining that the child is unresponsive, check their breathing. If they are barely breathing or only gasping, begin CPR. Gasping maybe forceful or weak, but it is generally ineffective. This is abnormal and often occurs in cardiac arrest.

If you are alone and must leave the child to activate EMS, give five sets of compressions and breaths (about two minutes) before leaving the child. (The AHA points out that most rescuers are likely to have speakerphone equipped cell phones, so the rescuer can call 911 without leaving the child) *(Figure 22c)*.

>> Next: Choking in Children

CHOKING IN CHILDREN

Choking can be mild or severe. If the child can make sounds and cough, the airway is mildly blocked. Stand near them and encourage them to cough. Call 911 immediately if you are worried about their breathing.

Severe signs of blockage include the inability to breathe, coughing without making a sound, inability to speak, or the universal choking sign. In any of these cases, immediate action is required.

Table 2 will help determine whether the choking is mild or severe.

DEGREE OF OBSTRUCTION	CHILD'S RESPONSE	RESCUER'S ACTIONS
Mild Obstruction	• *breathing but may also be wheezing* • *coughing and making noise*	• *stay with the child and try to keep them calm* • *call 911 if the obstruction is not cleared quickly*
Severe Obstruction	• *weak or no cough* • *unable to make noise or makes high-pitched noise* • *little or no breathing* • *appears cyanotic (blue around lips and fingertips)*	• *act fast* • *follow the steps for relief of choking for child*

Table 2

>> Next: Relief of Choking

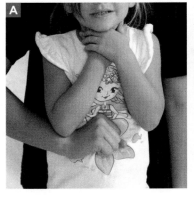
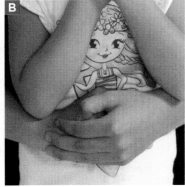
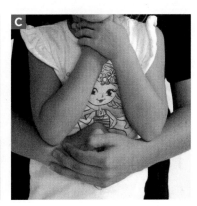

Figure 24:
Heimlich Maneuver

RELIEF OF CHOKING

Use the Heimlich maneuver learned in the adult section for children who are choking.

To relieve choking in a child, do the following:

1. Ask if they are choking.
2. Tell them you will help.
3. Stand behind them and wrap your arms around their body below the rib cage *(Figure 24a)*.
4. Make a fist with one hand and place it just above the navel *(Figure 24b)*.
5. Grab the fist with your other hand and deliver quick upward thrusts *(Figure 24c)*.
6. Continue until the obstruction comes out and breathing is possible, coughing or speaking is restored, or until the child stops responding.

If you can see a foreign object in the child's mouth and can easily remove it, do so. Avoid blindly sweeping the mouth with a finger as it may push the object deeper into the airway. Watch and feel for breathing to begin. If the child does not respond or begin breathing, begin CPR and continue to provide it until additional help arrives.

Large children may require chest thrusts if you cannot wrap your arms fully around the waist. In this case, perform the Heimlich maneuver with your fist on the breastbone.

Any child who has had a severe choking event should see a doctor.

If the child stops responding, lay them down and yell for help. Check for breathing and begin CPR. After 30 compressions, open the airway and look for a foreign object. If visible, remove it and attempt to give a breath. Continue CPR until the child recovers or more advanced help arrives.

>> Next: Self-Assessment for Child CPR, AED and Choking

SELF-ASSESSMENT FOR CHILD CPR, AED AND CHOKING

1. What is the main difference in care when finding an unresponsive adult versus an unresponsive child if you must leave the person to activate EMS?

    a. There is no difference.
    b. Perform CPR first when with an adult; go for help first when with a child.
    c. Perform two minutes of CPR when with a child, then go for help; call for help immediately when with an adult.
    d. It depends on the age of the child.

2. You are a daycare provider and find a three-year-old child unresponsive. She had laid down for a nap because she was not feeling well. When you checked on her, she was not breathing and appeared blue. You are by yourself. What is the first step in managing this case?

    a. Do back blows.
    b. Do a blind finger sweep.
    c. Call 911.
    d. Deliver two minutes of CPR.

3. You are concerned that a child may have choked. What is the best method to clear a foreign object from the airway?

    a. Heimlich maneuver
    b. CPR
    c. Back blows/ chest thrusts
    d. Blind finger sweep

4. You are performing CPR on a six-year-old child. The AED arrives. Which of the following is most appropriate?

    a. Use adult pads.
    b. Use pediatric pads.
    c. AED cannot be used on a six-year-old.
    d. Wait for EMS to arrive.

>> Next: Self-Assessment Answers

ANSWERS

1. C
   When coming upon an unresponsive child who requires CPR, deliver five sets of compressions and breaths before going for help. For an adult requiring CPR, call for help immediately and then return to the person to begin CPR.

2. D
   If you are alone, unwitnessed arrest in a child requires two minutes of CPR before activating EMS. If assistance is available, send to call 911 while you begin CPR.

3. B
   Chest compressions are delivered to the unresponsive during CPR. The AHA recommends to do chest compressions without a pulse check in the child who becomes unresponsive in a choking emergency.

4. B
   Pediatric pads should be used when available. If using adult pads, make sure they do not touch each other. Do not delay the use of an AED.

>> Next: Infant CPR and Choking

7

INFANT CPR AND CHOKING

Infants more often have a breathing problem than an actual heart problem. Prevention of choking in infants is crucial. It is important to begin CPR immediately and perform five sets of CPR before going to get additional help.

If someone else is available, send them to call 911 and to find an AED. One set of CPR consists of 30 compressions and two breaths. When the second rescuer returns, have them follow the AED prompts, apply AED pads, and help with CPR.

If the infant is unresponsive and not breathing or only gasping for air, provide CPR.

When giving CPR to an infant victim, do the following:

1. Make sure the scene and area around the infant is safe.
2. Tap and shout to determine if the infant is unresponsive.
3. Yell for help. If a second person is available have them call 911 and get an AED.
4. Check breathing.
5. If not responding and not breathing or only gasping, then give five sets of 30 compressions and two breaths.
6. Call 911 if a second person has not already done so.
7. Resume CPR and give compressions and breaths.

INFANT CPR (0 TO 12 MONTHS)

CPR for children and infants is almost identical. An infant that does nothing when you tap or talk loudly is considered unresponsive and CPR needs to be given.

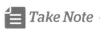 *Take Note*

As a rescuer, if you are untrained in CPR, then give the "hands-only" CPR. The "hands-only" CPR is when you give continuous compressions but no breaths.

>> Next: Compressions

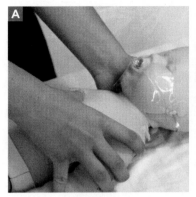
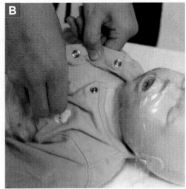
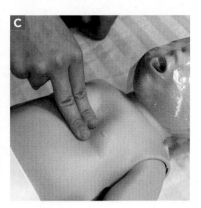

Figure 25

COMPRESSIONS

Push hard and fast as you would in a child or adult receiving CPR. Position the infant on a firm, hard surface to make giving CPR easier.

To give an infant CPR, do the following:

1. Position the infant on their back on a firm, hard surface *(Figure 25a)*.
2. Move any clothing away from the chest *(Figure 25b)*.
3. Place two fingers of one hand on the breastbone right below the nipple line *(Figure 25c)*.
4. Push straight down approximately 1.5 inches (4 cm) at a rate of 100 to 120 beats per minute.
5. Let the chest recoil to its normal position after every compression.

Performing compressions correctly is essential to effective CPR and can be physically tiring. If someone else can help, switch off every two minutes while minimizing interruptions during compressions.

>> Next: Giving Breaths

GIVING BREATHS

Giving breaths during CPR can help infants. Like children, many cases of cardiac arrest in infants are primarily due to respiratory problems. Giving breaths and administering chest compressions are important for infants receiving CPR. A good breath will cause the chest to rise.

To open the infant's airway, do the following:

1. Put one hand on the forehead.

2. Place your fingers on the bony part of the chin.

3. Gently tilt the head back while lifting the chin.

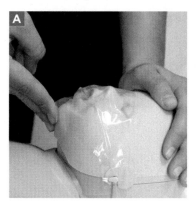 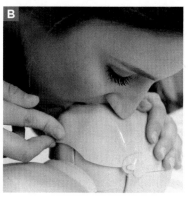 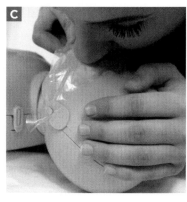

Figure 26

Be careful not to tilt the head too far back as this can block the airway. Be sure to press on the bony part of the chin and not the soft part under the chin as pressing the soft part may also block the airway.

Once you've opened the infant's airway, you are ready to give breaths. Next, do the following:

1. Hold the airway open as described above by gently pressing forehead back and lifting chin with your fingers. *(Figure 26a)*.

2. Take a deep breath and seal your mouth around the infant's mouth and nose *(Figure 26b)*.

3. Blow for one second and watch the chest rise *(Figure 26c)*. Very little volume or force is required to inflate an infant's lungs. Blowing too much or too hard will damage the infant's lungs. Only a gentle exhale for a tiny puff of air is required for an infant.

4. Repeat for a second breath.

If unable to cover both mouth and nose entirely with your mouth, use the following method for rescue breathing:

1. Open the airway using the head-tilt/chin-lift maneuver.

2. Pinch the infant's nose closed. Create a seal using your lips to surround the infant's mouth.

If the chest does not rise after the first breath, let the head go back to normal position and then re-open the airway by tilting head and lifting the chin. Try to get a breath in while watching for chest rise. Do not interrupt compressions for any more than 10 seconds when giving breaths.

>> Next: Mask Use

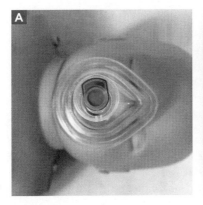 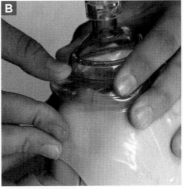 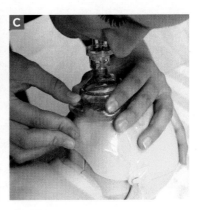

Figure 27

MASK USE

Giving breaths in CPR is generally safe for the rescuer. However, if a mask is available, it should be used. The mask fits over the infant's mouth and nose. Many masks have a pointed or tapered end which should go over the bridge of the infant's nose. Make sure the mask fits properly; if it is too large, a proper seal cannot be obtained and efforts to deliver breaths will be ineffective.

When using a mask to give breaths, do the following:

1. Place the mask over the infant's mouth and nose *(Figure 27a)*.

2. Open the airway by performing the head-tilt/chin-lift maneuver.

3. Ensure a good seal between the mask and the face *(Figure 27b)*.

4. Give a breath over one second and watch the chest rise *(Figure 27c)*.

ACTIVATING EMS (CALLING 911)

1. Always make sure the scene is safe when approaching an infant. If you become injured or disabled, it will only make the situation worse.

2. Tap the infant and talk loudly to determine if they are unresponsive. If they fail to make any response or reaction, they are considered unresponsive. An unresponsive infant will not move when you touch them. They will not cry or make any sounds, and their body will be limp.

3. Yell for help and call 911 using a cell phone. If no cell phone is available, send someone else to call 911 if possible.

4. If you are alone, begin five cycles of CPR (about two minutes) before calling 911.

>> Next: Choking in Infants

CHOKING IN INFANTS

Choking occurs when food or a foreign object is stuck in the throat and blocks the airway. Infants often put small objects in their mouth and are at an increased risk of choking. Severe choking requires quick action. Immediately perform back slaps and chest thrusts.

Table 3 will help determine whether the choking is mild or severe.

DEGREE OF OBSTRUCTION	INFANT'S RESPONSE	RESCUER'S ACTIONS
Mild Obstruction	• *breathing but may also be wheezing* • *coughing and making noise*	• *stay with the infant and try to keep them calm* • *call 911 if the obstruction is not cleared quickly*
Severe Obstruction	• *weak or no cough* • *unable to make noise; or makes high-pitched noise* • *little or no breathing* • *appears cyanotic (blue around lips and fingertips)*	• *act fast* • *follow the steps for relief of choking for infant*

Table 3

>> Next: Choking in Infants

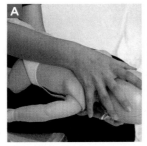
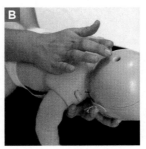
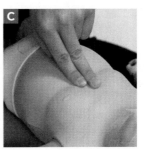
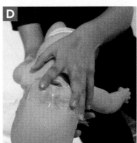

Figure 28

RELIEF OF CHOKING

Back slaps and chest thrusts are used on infant who are choking.

When an infant is choking, do the following:

1. Hold the infant in your lap.
2. Put the infant face down and the head lower than the chest; the infant should be resting on your forearm. Put your forearm on your thigh *(Figure 28a)*.
3. Support the infant's head and neck with your hand and be sure to avoid putting pressure on the throat.
4. Give five back slaps between the infant's shoulder blades with the heel of your hand. *(Figure 28b)*.
5. Using both hands and arms, turn the infant face up, so they are now resting on your other arm; this arm should now be resting on your thigh.
6. Using two fingers in the same spot as for CPR, provide five quick chest thrusts *(Figure 28c)*.
7. If the obstruction is not relieved, turn the infant face down on your other forearm and repeat the process. *(Figure 28d)*.
8. Continue until the infant begins to breathe or becomes unresponsive.

Try to keep the infant's head lower than the rest of the body when performing back slaps and chest thrusts. If you can see a foreign object in the infant's mouth and can easily remove it, do so. Avoid blindly sweeping the mouth with a finger as it may push a foreign object deeper into the airway. Watch and feel for breathing to begin.

If the infant stops responding, position them on a firm, flat surface and yell for help. Check for breathing and begin CPR. After 30 compressions, open the airway and look for a foreign object. If visible, remove it and attempt to ventilate with two breaths.

If the infant does not respond or begin breathing, continue to provide CPR until additional help arrives. You will know an infant has become unresponsive as they will stop moving and squirming in your arms and the body will become limp. In this case, begin CPR immediately with chest compressions followed by giving breaths.

>> Next: Self-Assessment for Infant CPR and Choking

SELF-ASSESSMENT FOR INFANT CPR AND CHOKING

1. The generally accepted age of an infant is less than:
    a. one year old
    b. two years old
    c. three years old
    d. four years old

2. You are attempting to relieve choking in an infant. The infant now becomes unresponsive. What is the next step?
    a. Leave the infant to get help.
    b. Do a blind finger sweep.
    c. Begin CPR.
    d. Do abdominal thrusts.

3. What is the most common cause of cardiac arrest in infants?
    a. Heart problems
    b. Respiratory problems
    c. Diabetes
    d. Poisoning

4. You come across an infant who is not responsive. When should you call 911?
    a. Immediately
    b. After five cycles (two minutes) of CPR
    c. After giving two breaths
    d. After 30 chest compressions

ANSWERS

1. A
    Infants are considered to be less than one year of age. A child is between one year and puberty.

2. C
    If an infant becomes unresponsive during attempt to relieve choking, position them on a firm, flat surface and begin CPR.

3. B
    Respiratory problems usually precede cardiac arrest in both infants and children.

4. B
    Give five cycles of 30 compressions and two breaths in an unresponsive infant before going to call 911. If someone is available to help, send them immediately to call 911.

>> Next: Additional Tools

8 ADDITIONAL TOOLS

MEDICODE

With MediCode, you no longer will have to carry a set of expandable cards with you at all times while at work. You will never have to waste valuable time in an emergency situation searching through multiple algorithms until you find the right one. All of the algorithms are now accessible from the palm of your hand, and you will be selecting your desired algorithm by memory in no time. Choose between multiple viewing options and easily share algorithms with co-workers and friends through email and social media.

To improve functionality and speed in obtaining your desired algorithm as quickly as possible in an emergency, they have been divided between BLS, ACLS , PALS and CPR. All are accessible from the home screen. The individual algorithms included within this app are:

- Basic Life Support (BLS)
- Advanced Cardiac Life Support (ACLS)
- Pediatric Advanced Life Support (PALS)
- Cardiopulmonary Resuscitation (CPR) AED, and First Aid

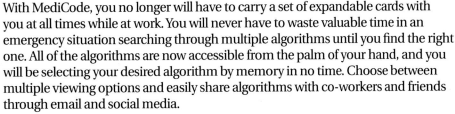

CERTALERT+

CertAlert+ is the perfect app to minimize a potential area of stress and distraction in your life. With CertAlert+, you will have all your licenses and certifications in one place anytime you need them. We will keep track and remind you when your expiration date approaches, and we will help you with your registration whenever possible.

With CertAlert+, you can:

- Compile all required licenses and certifications in one location.
- Take photos (front and back) of certification cards and licenses for simple reference.
- Record all expiration dates and store with ease.
- Choose when you want to be reminded of your approaching expiration dates.
- Send all license or certification information directly to your email after exporting from the app.
- Quick access to easily register for online certification and recertification courses.

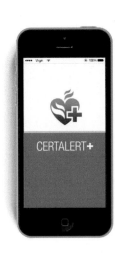

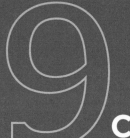

1. CPR steps are:

   a. Airway, Breathing, Check pulse
   b. Compressions, Airway, Breathing
   c. Airway, Breathing, Compressions
   d. Airway, Check pulse, Breathing

2. Critical characteristics of high-quality CPR include which of the following?

   a. Starting chest compressions within 10 seconds of recognition of cardiac arrest
   b. Allowing complete chest recoil after each compression
   c. Minimizing interruptions of CPR
   d. All of the above

3. At what age is it necessary to use the child AED pads if available?

   a. 17
   b. 16
   c. 14
   d. Up until puberty

4. The compression to ventilation ratio for the one-rescuer CPR for any age is:

   a. 30:1
   b. 30:2
   c. 15:1
   d. 15:2

5. Where on an adult requiring CPR should chest compressions be delivered?

   a. On the upper half of the breastbone
   b. On the lower half of the breastbone
   c. On the center of the chest
   d. Over the abdomen

6. An AED can be used safely in all of the following situations except:

   a. Person lying in the snow
   b. Person with an implanted pacemaker
   c. Person with a transdermal medication patch on
   d. Person lying partially in water

7. You are alone when you encounter a person in what appears to be cardiac or respiratory arrest. What are the first three steps you should take to stabilize the person? Check for danger, _____, and send for help.

   a. Establish IV access
   b. Insert an advanced airway
   c. Check for response
   d. Start CPR

8. What is the proper depth of chest compressions for adults during CPR?

    a. 1 to 2 inches
    b. 2 to 2.4 inches
    c. 4 to 5 inches
    d. More than 6 inches

9. The proper steps for operating an AED are:

    a. Power on the AED, attach electrode pads, shock the person, and analyze the rhythm
    b. Power on the AED, attach electrode pads, analyze the rhythm, and shock the person
    c. Power on the AED, analyze the rhythm, attach electrode pads, and shock the person
    d. Power on the AED, shock the person, attach electrode pads, and analyze the rhythm

10. What is the preferred method to relieve choking in infants?

    a. Finger sweep
    b. Abdominal thrusts
    c. Back slaps and chest thrusts
    d. Back slaps only

ANSWERS

1. B
   Compressions, Airway, Breathing

2. D
   All of the above

3. D
   Use pediatric pads for persons who have not yet reached puberty.

4. B
   30:2

5. C
   CPR is delivered in the center of the chest on the lower half of the breastbone but above the xyphoid process.

6. D
   Person lying partially in water

7. C
   Check for response.

8. B
   2 to 2.4 inches

9. B
   Power on the AED, attach electrode pads, analyze the rhythm, and shock the patient

10. C
    Back slaps and chest thrusts 2 to 2.4 inches

Made in the USA
Columbia, SC
28 December 2018